Essential Oils

A Better Health Guide to Essential Oils for Stress Relief, Weight Loss, Vitality, and Longevity

KARA AIMER

ISBN: **1512219355**
ISBN-13: **978-1512219357**

CONTENTS

INTRODUCTION

We all have moments when we are stressed such that we feel as if our world is tearing apart. What do you do in such moments? Do you sleep for stress management? Do you travel or do yoga or even exercise to get some relief? Or do you opt to eat or drink until you pass out then wake up the next day feeling all crappy and hating yourself?

Well, whatever method you use, I must say that something that has continually worked for me is aromatherapy. Simply inhaling the essential oils brings me a feeling of overwhelming relief. The amazing thing about essential oils is that they are not only useful in relieving stress but also in treating various ailments as well as in helping you lose weight.

This book will look closely at what essential oils are, their role in stress relief as well as in treating other conditions, and how to use the essential oils because there are various ways to use them other than just inhaling them. You will also learn how to specifically use them in order to achieve whatever goals you have in mind

WHAT ARE ESSENTIAL OILS AND CARRIER OILS?

Essential Oils

An essential oil refers to the liquid that is usually distilled (by water or steam) from the roots, bark, flowers, stems, leaves and many other elements of a plant. The oil is essential in the sense that it contains the characteristic fragrance of the plant from which it is derived. This doesn't mean that essential oils are the same as fragrance or perfume oils.

These two are very different in that essential oils are obtained from true plants while perfume oils are usually artificially created fragrances that don't have any therapeutic benefits that are offered by essential oils. Actually, the chemical composition and the aroma of essential oils have different physical and psychological therapeutic benefits. For you to obtain these benefits you can use the essential oils through application of the diluted oil to your skin or through inhalation; there are instances when you can use the oil through ingestion although this has to be done with instructions from a doctor.

Essential oils are generally extracted by distillation, expression, or solvent extraction. Some common examples of essential oils include:

Bitter Almond Essential Oil – This is traditionally used as a diuretic, germicide, fungicide, sedative, anesthetic, anti-oxidant, and a cure for hydrophobia.

Birch Essential Oil – This is a stimulant, disinfectant, analgesic, detoxifier, germicide, insecticide and depurative.

Anise Essential Oil – This is used as an anti-epileptic, antiseptic, antihysteric, anti-rheumatic, decongestant, digestive, stimulant and sedative.

Angelica Essential Oil – This can be used as an anti-spasmodic, diuretic, hepatic, expectorant, stomachic and tonic.

Basil Essential Oil – This is used as an analgesic, anti-bacterial, ophthalmic, carminative and anti-spasmodic.

Black Pepper Essential Oil – This is used as a digestive, anti-rheumatic, anti-bacterial and anti-oxidant.

Other common essential oils include lavender, cardamom, carrot seed, celery, clove, clary sage, jasmine, juniper, lemongrass, lime, marjoram, oregano, orange, peppermint, rose, sage, tarragon, wintergreen and ylang ylang. The list of essential oils is quite long. Here is a comprehensive list of essential oils.

It would be wrong to talk about the use of essential oils without mentioning carrier oils. So, what are carrier oils and what do they do? Let's take a closer look.

Carrier Oils

Carrier oils, also known as base/vegetable oils, are derived from the fatty portion of plants. They are used to dilute essential oils before applying on the skin especially given the fact that essential oils are highly concentrated in their undiluted form. Carrier oils are named so because they carry essential oils to the skin. This doesn't mean that they are all equal in various properties. For instance, they usually vary in their viscosities. Some examples of carrier oils include:

Avocado Oil – This is thick in texture and leaves a fatty and almost waxy feel to the skin. It has a medium aroma, somewhat sweet and nut.

Borage Oil – It has a sweet and light aroma. It has a thin-medium texture, somewhat oily on the skin.

Calendula Oil – This is yellow to amber in color, thin in texture and has a spicy-sweet aroma.

Cocoa Butter – The aroma is very sweet and rich of chocolate, in the case of unrefined cocoa butter. It is tan in color and solid at room temperature.

Coconut Oil – This is light in color, has coconut aroma and is easy to spread and non-oily.

Sweet Almond Oil – It has nutty, slightly sweet and light aroma. It is almost completely clear with a trace of yellow in color. It absorbs moderately leaving the skin feeling lightly oily. It is considered all-purpose carrier oil.

Olive Oil – It smells like olives and has a heavy and oily texture. The greener the oil, the closer it is to pure cold pressed. You may blend 10% of it with other carrier oil.

Jojoba Oil – It has a light to nearly odorless aroma. It has a silky texture and usually absorbs well into the skin although it can feel waxy. It is yellow in color and does not go rancid very quickly.

Macadamia Nut Oil – It has a very sweet and very aromatic aroma than any other nut oils. Because of its thickness, it leaves an oily film on the skin. It is clear with a slightly yellow hue in color.

Peanut Oil – This has a light with a slightly nutty aroma. It is thick in texture and very oily on the skin. It is not suitable for anyone with an allergy to peanuts.

Pecan Oil – It has an extremely light and nutty aroma. Its texture is medium and it is slightly oily on the skin. It is clear in color and has a possibility of turning rancid quickly.

Other carrier oils include Watermelon Seed Oil, Sunflower Oil, Sesame Oil, Rose Hip Oil, Pomegranate Oil, Kukui Nut Oil, Hazel Nut Oil, Grape Seed Oil, and Apricot Kernel Oil.

So how do you purchase the best essential oil for whatever use you want it for?

ESSENTIAL OILS BUYING GUIDE

Below are some important tips that will come in handy when purchasing essential oils:

1. Avoid buying essential oils from suppliers who don't provide the essentials oil's botanical name, method of extraction and the country of origin. The country of origin is important because the soils and climate conditions affect the resulting properties of the essential oil.

2. Find out which oil best suits your needs: You can ask your knowledgeable friends, herbalist or even research online. If you find out more than one option, eliminate by their prices.

3. Learn about the oil that you want to purchase: The more you can learn about the product, the better the value you will be able to get. For example, which parts of the plant were used, what was the method of extraction, the country, or region of its origin and the time of harvest? These factors affect the final quality of the oils.

4. Consider how oils are stored: Oils should be protected from excess heat or direct sunlight by storage in dark glass bottles or stainless steel containers. Shopping locally can help you see how oils are stored.

5. Find out about the manufacturer: Research the company that manufactures the oils that you are considering. Certain companies have a reputation of manufacturing quality products. Go for those.

6. Get an idea of the going prices: Check out for the best price of the product you have chosen; whether online or locally, the price should be

within a certain range. If you find a choice falling far below the range, there could be something fishy about the product.

7. If you are buying oils locally, watch out for dusty bottle tops. It indicates that the oils have been sitting around for a while. Oils oxidize with time and lose their therapeutic properties. Their aroma also diminishes.

8. It is not wise to purchase essential oils from a food store. Normally, they have more risk of oxidizing since they don't sell very quickly. In addition, the brands will be of low quality because of less optimal ways of storage.

9. When choosing to try a particular vendor, place a small order and ask for additional samples. This will help you find out if you are pleased with it without wasting your money on a large order that might not impress you.

10. Buying essential oils online gives you the opportunity to shop with many more reputable companies than being limited to your locale. Reputable companies are known for properly bottling and packaging their oils for shipment.

Before we can get into detail on how to use the various essential oils, it is important to look at some safety guidelines that will ensure you enjoy the benefits of essential oils and not put your health at risk.

SAFETY USE OF ESSENTIAL OILS

Below are some important guidelines that you have to follow as you start using essential oils.

1. Ensure you use essential oils in a well-ventilated room, as excessive inhalation of essential oils could be unhealthy.

2. Keep essential oils away from direct flame such as candles, cooking gas and matches since they are highly flammable.

3. Do not use any essential oils internally unless you are certain about its safe internal use. You should also have been trained on safety issues relating to internal use. Should you accidentally ingest any significant amount of essential oil, contact the nearest poison control unit. Do not induce vomiting.

4. Keep essential oils away from eyes. In case a drop finds its way into the eye, use a cotton piece of cloth imbued with fatty oil to swipe over the closed lid. Alternatively, flush the eyes immediately with cool water.

5. In the case of pregnancy, old age or a serious health issue, do not use essential oils before doing an advanced medical study and seeking the advice of your doctor.

6. Perform a skin patch test first before using the essential oil to ascertain whether you are allergic to certain essential oils.

7. Avoid using undiluted essential oils on the skin unless stated

otherwise. Essential oils are very concentrated and could be irritating to the skin. Dilute all essential oils in carrier oils before applying to the skin.

8. Avoid the prolonged use of the same essential oils, as this can make your body be resistant to the essential oils, which means that you may not enjoy some benefits that a particular essential oil offers.

9. Discontinue the use of the essential oils that cause dermal irritation. Apply vegetable oil or cream to the affected area.

10. Keep all essentials out of reach of children and pets to avoid accidents.

11. Do not use photosensitizing essential oils before you go out in the sun. Photosensitizing occurs when an agent or certain essential oils, in our case, are used causing the skin to be more sensitive to the sunlight or any UV light causing it to be damaged or to burn more easily. Examples of essential oils that are phototoxic are; cold pressed bitter orange, bergamot, lemon, cold pressed grapefruit, orange, and tangerine.

In the following chapters, we will look at various essential oils for stress relief, for weight loss and for treating various ailments.

ESSENTIAL OILS FOR STRESS RELIEF

As earlier indicated, I especially love essential oils for stress relief. Below are some essential oils that you can use to relieve stress.

Lavender
It has a calming, earthy, lightly sweet, and freshly floral scent. It is well known for its balancing and relaxing effects on both the physical body and emotions. It is able to do this because the lavender plant is rich in linalyl acetate and linalool, which has been proven to cross the blood-brain barrier. This will leave you feeling relaxed and sharper. In addition to stress relief, it also helps in anxiety relief and short-memory enhancement.

Since it can be safely used directly on your skin, you can rub 2-3 drops and massage them on your temple. You can also choose to apply a few drops on the palm of your hand and inhale deeply.

Lemon Balm
This herb is commonly used to help with stress, anxiety, and insomnia. Lemon does not only calm your mind but also improves your ability to concentrate and solve problems.

To use it, just apply 3-4 drops of high-quality lemon balm on the palms of your hands and inhale deeply for 30 seconds.

Frankincense
This oil has a very warm and exotic aroma that has a relaxing effect on the human body. This includes uplifting your mood and heightening awareness. To apply this, dilute several drops of frankincense with carrier oil and rub on shoulders, neck, and spine.

Rose Geranium

Rose geranium has a very great flowery scent. It has the ability to relax your entire body as well as boost your mood if you are feeling down. This plant has been found to balance hormonal levels and even provide a major boost of relaxation and less irritability.

Upon smelling it, it provides a soothing sensation to the entire central nervous system. It can take away pain throughout the body, and stimulate the lymphatic system.

Roman Chamomile

The smell of this oil is distinguishable from other scents. It smells a little sweet or fruity at times. The oil is usually obtained from the chamomile flowers.

Roman chamomile oil has been established to reduce stress, insomnia and muscle tension. It works primarily by having a calming effect on the user. Because of this, it can help with a variety of ailments including vomiting and restlessness. Applying it on the skin can help to soothe any tension within the muscles.

Bergamot

The actual oil is usually derived from the rind of unripe citrus fruit from a bitter orange tree. The scent is helpful at restoring the hypothalamus to a state of calmness inducing a state of relaxation. The oil can be administered by sniffing directly from the bottle or by rubbing a drop or two on the palm of your hand.

Jasmine

Jasmine oil is extracted from the plant's flowers. It is usually picked in the evening to maximize on fragrance. This oil has a wonderful aroma that relieves stress by making you feel happy and potentially awakens romantic and poetic feeling. The romantic effect of jasmine helps stimulate the release of certain hormones in the body including serotonin, which results in the boost of energy and uplifted mood.

Jasmine oil is just as strong and good as valium, an anti-anxiety drug. It works by increasing the GABA activity in the brain to help regulate feelings of stress and anxiety. You can put several drops of jasmine oil on the palm of your hand and then inhale deeply.

Sandalwood

This essential oil is clear and appears to have a slightly yellowish tint. Sandalwood oil creates a harmonizing and calming effect for the mind helping reduce confusion and tension.

Sweet Marjoram

This bold fragrance has a little spice, but it still leads to a state of relaxation of mind and body. It also helps with insomnia problems. You can inhale the aroma from the bottle for a calming effect. It is best used in combination with other essential oils like bergamot and chamomile for an even more powerful effect.

In addition to single essential oils that you can use to get relief from stress, you may also want to try different blends or essential oils, which are likely to yield maximum results. Below are two main blends for stress relief:

Balancing Blend

This is a blend of blue chamomile, blue tansy, frankincense, hop wood, and spruce. The oils in this blend are geared towards the central nervous system. This blend is a great option when you are feeling unsettled, anxious, doubtful, confused, or stressed. It is a perfect choice when dealing with temper problems, unsettled emotions, or mood swings. If you wear a clay necklace, apply some on it and inhale the fragrance all day.

Elevation Blend

This blend consists of tangerine, ilang-ilang, sandalwood, osmanthus, Melissa, lavender, clemi and lemon myrtle.

The blend addresses issues with stress, depression, attention, hopelessness, fatigue, and anxiety. You simply breathe in this oil directly from the bottle and breathe out your worries.

ESSENTIAL OILS FOR WEIGHT LOSS

Are you aware that you can actually lose weight by simply making use of essential oils? Let us have a look at some amazing essential oils that you can use for weight loss.

Grapefruit

This oil is the best for weight loss because of the d-limonene found in grapefruit. D-limonene helps you lose weight by lowering cholesterol and reducing lipid peroxidation. D-limonene is also known for its many health benefits like fat burning, lymphatic system detox, and metabolism stimulation.

As you are aware, toxicity in the body creates unwanted weight gain. Grapefruit essential oil releases these toxins from our metabolic pathway. Grapefruit oil also has anti-oxidant properties and anti-inflammatory uses along with natural weight loss management properties.

You can add 1-2 drops of grapefruit essential oil to your drinking water to flush out toxins and for its fat burning effects, especially before breakfast in the morning.

Peppermint

Peppermint is great for reducing appetite and suppression of cravings. It is able to suppress appetite as it works on that part of the brain that triggers the feeling of fullness. It also helps with treating candida, which often influences weight gain and management. In addition, this oil is packed with minerals like magnesium, iron, and potassium and nutrients like vitamin C and omega-3-fatty acids. Therefore, in addition to weight loss maintenance, it also nourishes the body and promotes a feeling of well-being.

You can add 1-2 drops in a glass of drinking water and enjoy the drink.

Lemon

Just like peppermint, inhaling lemon essential oil scent is a natural way to control appetite therefore helping in weight loss. Lemon essential oil also contains d-limonene and it's full of vitamins and minerals. This makes it great for fighting intestinal parasites, which have been proven to be a major contributor of weight gain.

It also helps in weight loss by fighting various digestive ailments, increasing energy levels and balancing metabolism. It helps the body carry fewer toxins, which it stores in the fat cells.

You can use this oil by rubbing it on the cellulite areas. This helps to eliminate wastes and toxins that are stored in the fat cells. This rids the body of these toxins, making you thinner and healthier. You can also choose to inhale lemon essential oil before meals.

Bergamot

Bergamot oil contains large amounts of polyphenol, which is great for fat oxidation, preventing absorption of cholesterol and increasing metabolism. This makes it effective for weight control.

Bergamot also inhibits an enzyme that is linked to blood sugar levels. It becomes more active when sugar is high which promotes the decomposition of sugar and fats. Additionally, this oil is perfect if you have an emotional eating problem. If paired with lavender oil, the two exhibit great sedative properties making them perfect to fight stress related weight gain and controlling stress triggered eating.

You can also use bergamot by mixing it with carrier oil then massaging your feet or your neck. You can also put a few drops on a cloth and inhale the vapors to calm and relax when you are stressed and tempted to eat more.

Cinnamon Bark

It works more as a weight gain preventer and less as a weight loss remedy. This essential oil gives you a feeling of fullness after meals. This is because it helps in breaking down the sugar for absorption into the body as energy. This then results in less fatty acids being stored. Cinnamon also helps in increasing blood circulation, improving gut health, treating irritable bowel syndrome, and increasing metabolism as well as stimulating the immune system. This makes it helpful in weight management. It is also found to be effective in getting rid of candida, which influences weight gain.

Combine a few drops of cinnamon essential oil with honey in a glass of water then drink before sleeping and before breakfast. You can also inhale cinnamon essential oil before meals.

Sandalwood Essential Oil
Sandalwood essential oil, just like bergamot oil, works well in stress eating. It helps overcome negative feelings and behavior so that you don't feel tempted to eat more in the name of dealing with stress.

You can diffuse it and inhale the vapors by diluting it in a ratio of 1:1 with the carrier oil. You can also apply it directly on the stomach or to the feet.
Other essential oil blends that are perfect for helping in weight loss include:

Endocrine Essential Oil Blend
This essential oil blend helps to support the endocrine system i.e. the thyroid and maintain overall vitality. It is a blend of German chamomile, myrtle, geranium, sage and seed oil as the carrier oil. Endocrine essential oil blend helps in increasing metabolism, improving circulation and promoting the healthy production of enzymes in the body.

To use it, apply 1-2 drops topically over the lower back for kidney, liver and kidneys.

Stress Away Blend
This is an essential oil blend made with vanilla, Ocotea, lime, lavender, cedar wood, copaiba, and cedar wood. It is effective in combating stress, restoring equilibrium and relieving occasional nervous tension. The vanilla oil in the blend can help to curb sweet and chocolate cravings. The Ocotea in stress away blend may help to create a feeling of fullness and help to control hunger cravings.

To use this blend, put 2-3 drops of it in the palm of your hand and inhale for 30 seconds at a time, three times a day.

HEALING OF COMMON AILMENTS USING ESSENTIAL OILS

Essential oils are also very effective in treating various ailments. We will have a look at some common ailments and see how you can use essential oils to treat them.

Sore muscles
Black spruce essential oil is used to ease muscle tension. It is also great in reducing inflammation and soothing soreness. You could use it as your post workout remedy for recurring muscles aches or post workout soreness. You can also use it for lower back pain, sciatica and arthritis.

Apply 2-3 drops of this essential oil and gently rub on the affected area.

Cough or cold
Eucalyptus essential oil is ideal for colds and coughs because it has antibacterial, and antiviral properties. It helps in disinfecting and cleaning both lungs and the nasal passage.

You can add a few drops in a basin of steaming water to inhale. To prevent a full cold during a cold season, you can have a handkerchief in handy having a drop or two of eucalyptus essential oil.

Fatigue
Breathing in peppermint scent usually has a great energy giving effect. A whiff of it makes you feel fresh and peppy. The menthol in peppermint brings about an intense cool feeling. Ensure it is dilute before putting it on your skin because its concentration can be overwhelming for sensitive skin.

Place 1-2 drops on your palms, rub them together, and inhale during a midday slumber or before a workout.

Skin woes

Adding a small amount of rosehip essential oil into your facial cream helps to oxygenate and heal your skin. Rosehip essential oil has a high amount of fatty acids that are unsaturated, which can help generate cells of the membranes, minimize wrinkles and aging spots, slow the signs of aging, reduce scars and treat sun damaged skin.

Wounds

In the case of an infected wound, rashes, a burn or a cut, use Melrose oil. It will help in preventing infection, especially when the wound is open. It is also an excellent tissue generator and antiseptic. Before using it, dilute it in a 50:50 ratio with a carrier oil of your choice.

Lost concentration and Poor memory

Vetiver essential oil comes from the roots of a perennial grass and whose scent when inhaled, is likely to improve your concentration and memory. When you are about to head into a situation that requires heavy concentration or you are facing distractions, just apply 2-3 drops of it at the base of your neck or on your temples.

Insomnia

The lavender essential oil improves sleep since it makes the muscles relax and the heart beats slowly. At this point, the brain is thought to organize memory too. You can choose to diffuse a little in the room before going to sleep using an aromatherapy diffuser. You can also sprinkle a few drops on a cotton piece of cloth and tuck it under your pillow.

Headache and migraine pain

These two conditions are primarily triggered by stress. Therefore, relaxation is an important part of its treatment. Lavender oil has a calming effect and you can use it to treat headaches. You can rub it at the back of the neck or place a few drops into a glass of boiled water and inhale.

Nausea and vomiting

When you have nausea or you are vomiting, taking something orally is the last thing you will want to do. This makes, peppermint, ginger and nutmeg essential oils perfect for this job. They penetrate the skin and circulate through the body in a matter of minutes. Simply rub 2-3 drops of the respective essential oil over your stomach or colon to disperse them throughout your body.

Menstrual cramps

Marjoram oil is an analgesic that dilates blood vessels, which relieves menstrual cramps. It also has a component that interferes with prostaglandin pathway and has pain-relieving properties. Lavender and clary sage have one of the molecules that inhibit the secretion of prostaglandins that cause uterine muscle contraction.

Massage the abdominal area with one of these oils after dilution.

SKIN CARE WITH ESSENTIAL OILS

Essential oils are also amazing for dealing with different skin problems. Below are some essential oils and ways they can nourish your skin.

Lavender
In addition to its beautiful calming smell, lavender essential oil is a great disinfectant, which helps kill bacteria on your skin. It also heals wound and reduces redness. To use, mix 3 drops of jojoba oil and 1 drop of lavender oil on the palm of your hand and rub your palms together before applying to your face and neck.

Geranium
This oil is a great anti-inflammatory. It also helps to lighten overall skin tone and age spots. It also improves circulation under the skin surface, which aids in cell generation, making it useful for fading wrinkles, scars and other visible imperfections on the skin. Add 1-2 drops of geranium essential oil to your daily skin care routine.

Apricot Kernel
This oil is rich in omega 6-gamma linolenic acid, which helps to hydrate and nourish skin. Vitamin E contained in the oil encourages regeneration of skin cells and collagen production to help reduce wrinkles or fine lines. Kernel oil is used to hydrate and heal dry skin because the oil absorbs into skin relatively and quickly hence you can use it for massage.

Rosehip
This oil offers great properties of hydrating skin, reviving it instantly with a deeply penetrating level of moisture. It also improves skin elasticity, provides anti-aging properties, boosts skin cell regeneration, and reduces

scarring. Mix a few drops of rosehip oil with carrier oil and rub it on your face and neck.

Frankincense

Frankincense is effective in assisting in the generation of skin cells and keeps existing cells healthy, reducing the appearance of fine lines, wrinkles and appearance of scars. It is also great for tightening up sagging skin, balancing skin PH and evening skin tone.

Apply 2 drops of frankincense oil directly to the scars twice a day to help the spots fed.

Lemon Essential Oil

It can help lighten dark spots as well as prevent and reduce the appearance of wrinkles and lines. To use, add 3 drops of lemon essential oil to your daily skin moisturizer before applying.

Sandalwood

This oil can help fade scars, wrinkles, and lines as well as sooth damaged or irritated skin. For face oil and dry skin, add 4 drops of geranium and 8 drops sandalwood to sweet almond oil before using.

Cypress

Cypress oil can help reduce the appearance of varicose veins and broken capillaries under the skin surface. It also helps to strengthen skin and improve circulation. To treat varicose veins, mix 30 drops of cypress, 20 drops of lavender, 20 drops of lemongrass, and 10 drops of lemon with 60 drops of coconut oil.

ESSENTIAL OILS FOR HAIR CARE

If you want long, lustrous and healthy hair, essential oil is the way to go. Below are some essential oils you can use for hair care.

Carrot Root
Dilute carrot root with jojoba for use. It is rich in carotene and anti-oxidants that aid in hair growth.

Basil
It makes your hair oily and promotes growth by stimulating circulation.

Chamomile
Chamomile gives golden highlights and sheen to your hair. In addition to soothing an inflamed scalp, it also heals a scaly scalp and psoriasis as well as conditions your hair.

Cedar Wood
It is effective in treating hair loss and dandruff. It stimulates the scalp to normalize dry skin and oily scalp. It is also used as an antiseptic and astringent.

Eucalyptus
You can use it to treat dandruff and as an antiseptic.

Clary Sage
This can be used on all hair types to treat dandruff

Lavender

You can use this oil to balance natural scalp oils, to promote hair growth, soothe scalp, prevent hair breakage and calm hair. It also helps in scalp treatment for itchiness and dandruff.

Lemon
Lemon essential oil is effective in making hair oily. It also treats dry scalp and dandruff, lice and gives golden highlights. It also helps to balance natural scalp oils.

Lemon Grass
This essential oil is suitable for oily hair to slow down scalp oil production.

Myrrh
Myrrh is best for use on dry hair as a treatment for dry scalp and dandruff.

Tea tree
This is used in the treatment of dry scalp, dandruff, and lice. It is also a great moisturizer and helps to keep the scalp free of fungal and bacterial problems.

Thyme
This oil stimulates blood flow apart from being a great antiseptic.

Ylang-Ylang
This essential oil is amazing for stimulating hair growth, for the treatment of dandruff and for soothing the scalp. It is suitable for people with oily hair.

For conditioning
Use 3 drops of rosemary or any other essential oil
1 tablespoon of carrier oil
Mix the carrier oil and essential oil in a small dish. Wet your hair with warm water then apply the conditioner. Let it soak in for about 30 minutes then wash your hair as normal.

For scalp massage;
Place 3-5 drops of the hair conditioner oil from the recipe above on your fingertips and massage your scalp.

For scented hair;
Add 3 drops of hair care conditioner oil from the recipe above to your

hairbrush. As you comb your hair, the scent will be absorbed as the oil conditions your hair.

The next chapter will focus on some essential oil recipes that you can use.

ESSENTIAL OILS RECIPES

Emotional Wellbeing Recipes

Room air freshener recipe

Ingredients
1.5 fl. ounces distilled water or hydrosol
1.5 fl. ounces high proof alcohol - helps the aroma linger for a longer duration.
30-40 drops of essential oil of your choice
4 oz. spray bottle

Instructions
Fill the spray bottle with water and alcohol. Add the drops of essential oil and shake the bottle for a thorough mix. Let it sit for a day before using.

Shake the bottle immediately before each use. Mist the room lightly not allowing the mist to fall into open beverages or onto furniture.

Calming and relaxing recipe

Ingredients
5 drops lavender oil
7 drops roman chamomile essential oil
1 fl. ounce sweet almond oil

Instructions
Mix the oils and add to a clean airtight dark glass container.
Massage your feet with this relaxing oil to experience increased

calmness.

Insomnia blend

Ingredients
5 drops clary sage essential oil
5 drops bergamot essential oil
10 drops roman chamomile essential oil

Instructions
Blend all the oils well in a clean dark-colored glass bottle. Onto a piece of tissue, add about 2 drops of this oil and place inside a pillow. This will aid you in falling asleep.

Anxiety relieving recipe

Ingredients
1 drop vetiver oil
2 drops mandarin oil
1 drop lavender essential oil
1 drop rose oil

Instructions
Get 20 drops by multiplying the blend by 4. Add the oils into a dark colored glass bottle. Mix the contents well then follow manufacturer's instructions to add appropriate number of drops into your diffuser.

Energizing blend

Ingredients
2 drops lemon essence oil
1 drop frankincense oil
2 drops peppermint oil

Instructions
Obtain 20 drops by multiplying the blend by 4. Add the oils into a dark colored glass bottle and mix well. Add appropriate number of drops of your energizing blend to your diffuser and let it diffuse in the entire room.

Physical Wellbeing Recipes

Menstrual cramps recipe
Ingredients

3 drops lavender essential oil
4 drops Cyprus essential oil
5 drops peppermint essential oil
1 fl. Ounce jojoba

Instructions
Add all the oils into a clean, dark-colored glass bottle. Mix the oils evenly then gently massage a small amount into the abdominal area.

Sore muscles massage oil recipe

Ingredients
5 drops eucalyptus essential oil
4 drops peppermint essential oil
1 drop black pepper essential oil
2 drops ginger essential oil
1 fl. ounce sweet almond oil

Instructions
Add all the oils into an airtight, dark colored glass bottle. Mix them well to obtain an even mixture. Apply half a teaspoon on the affected muscle area for each massage.

Arthritis Recipe

Ingredients
4 drops black pepper essential oil
20 drops roman chamomile oil
2 fl. ounces sweet almond oil

Instructions
Put these oils in a small dish and blend them well. Store the mixture in an airtight dark-colored glass bottle. Put some on the palm of your hand and gently massage into arthritic joint.

Congestion Aromatherapy Blend
What you will need
Aromatherapy inhaler
4 drops peppermint essential oil
26 drops raven Sara essential oil
30 drops eucalyptus essential oil
Instructions
Blend the oils in a clean, dark-colored glass bottle. Put in an

aromatherapy inhaler then raise the inhaler to your nose and breathe deeply as needed.

Skincare, Beauty And Hygiene Recipes

Stretch marks recipe
What you will need
4 ounces jar with tight-fitting lid
4 drops of Neroli essential oil
1 fl. ounce Avocado oil
3 ounces cocoa butter

Instructions
Gently melt the cocoa butter in a double boiler. Stir in avocado oil and mix for a few minutes.

Pour the mixture into a small bowl and allow cooling for a couple of minutes before adding Neroli essential oil. Carefully pour the mixture into a jar after mixing.

Put a reasonable amount on the palms of your hand and apply to your upper thighs and abdomen at least twice a day.

Avoid genital areas and discontinue use if any sensitivity occurs.

Essential oil Shampoo Recipe

What you will need
8 oz. bottle
5 drops Ilang-ilang oil

10 drops rosemary oil
40 drops lavender oil
1 tablespoon jojoba oil
7 fl. ounces unscented shampoo base

Instructions
Add 7 fl. oz of unscented shampoo base to a mixing bowl. Blend in essential oils and mix well. Pour your shampoo into the 8 oz. bottle using a funnel.
Use the shampoo just like any other normal shampoo.

CONCLUSION

Essentials are not only good because of their amazing scents, they are also useful in healing a various of ailments, for healthy skin and hair as well as for helping you lose weight. If you want to experience better overall health, it is time to start using essential oils today.

Good luck, and congratulations on starting your path toward a happier, healthier, and more wholesome you!

Finally, if you enjoyed this book, please share your thoughts and post a positive review on Amazon. I would greatly appreciate your support!

Thank you and good luck!

Kara Aimer

ADDITIONAL RESOURCES

Please point your web browser to **www.plaid-enterprises.com** for more related resources, my full bibliography and to grab your FREE book!